Real Pregnancy Food For Women

The Knowledge And Science Behind Ideal Prenatal Nutrition

By

Beatrice Davis

Copyright © by Beatrice Davis 2023. All rights reserved

Real Pregnancy Food For Women

Table of content

Introduction   3
Chapter 1   6
Food and Food Classes   6
Chapter 2   11
What to Eat During Pregnancy: A Guide   11
Chapter 3   28
Foods That Foster Babies' Health   28
Chapter 4   35
Avoiding Certain Foods and Drinks While Pregnant35
Chapter 5   51
Nutritional Supplements   51

Introduction

The majority of women do not follow the guidelines for a healthy diet and weight before and during pregnancy. What a healthy pregnancy diet should look like is a question that both women and medical professionals frequently ask. The key phrase should be "Eat better, not more." This can be accomplished by replacing lower quality, highly processed meals with a variety of nutrient-dense, whole foods, such as fruits, vegetables, legumes, whole grains, and healthy fats with omega-3 fatty acids, which include nuts and seeds, and seafood.

A diet like this promotes nutritional density and is less prone than the typical diet, which includes increased intakes of processed foods, fatty red meat, and sweetened foods and beverages, to be accompanied by excessive energy intake. Pregnant women who report "prudent" or "health-conscious" eating habits may experience fewer pregnancy difficulties and un-unfavourable consequences for the health of their unborn children. Comprehensive nutritional supplementation (many micronutrients plus ll-balanced protein energy) has been linked to better pregnancy outcomes, including a decline in the incidence of low birth weight. The ketogenic diet, which excludes all carbs, the Paleo diet, which forbids the consumption of dairy products, and any diet with an excessive amount of saturated fats should all be avoided. It is vitally necessary to develop user-friendly solutions that allow for a quick assessment of dietary patterns, clear instructions on how to treat nutritional deficiencies, and embedded support from qualified healthcare professionals.

Recent research has revealed that whereas a high gestational weight increase among women of normal weight predicts negative perinatal outcomes, prepregnancy obesity predicts negative perinatal outcomes more strongly than gestational weight gain among women with obesity.

Chapter 1

Food and Food Classes

Any material that can support growth and development when ingested by a living organism is considered food. It controls potentially harmful or toxic substances from entering the body as well as the body's processes.

Categories of food

Food contains over 40 distinct types of nutrients, which can generally be divided into the following 7 major categories: carbs, proteins, fats, vitamins, minerals, dietary fibre, and water.

Although each of the seven primary nutrient groups has specific roles to play in our bodies, they are all necessary because they work together to support our overall health. The following list summarizes these important nutrients' main roles:

Carbohydrates

Our body uses carbohydrates, primarily found in grains like rice and noodles, as a key source of energy. In addition, carbs are found in fruit, root vegetables, dry beans, and dairy products.

Proteins

Good sources of protein include meat, fish, seafood, eggs, dairy products, dry beans, and bean products. Its primary duties include creating, maintaining, and repairing sound bodily tissues.

Fats

Meat, fish, seafood, dairy products, nuts, seeds, and oils are examples of foods that include fats. Fats are a source of energy. In extremely cold temperatures, they stop heat loss and save vital organs from shock. They are in charge of assembling some of the cells in our bodies and moving fat-soluble vitamins like vitamins A, D, E, and K.

Vitamins

Vitamins come in a wide variety and are found in a variety of dietary groups. They are involved in a variety of bodily processes, including bone development, keeping good skin and hair, and releasing and using energy from food. Vitamins can be divided into fat-soluble or water-soluble.

Minerals

Minerals are a class of important minerals that control a variety of bodily processes, including fluid equilibrium, muscle contraction, and nerve impulse transmission. Some elements, like calcium, support bone health and strength as well as body structure.

Consuming fibre

The component of plants that cannot be digested is called dietary fibre. It supports gastrointestinal health, prevents constipation, and stabilizes blood sugar. Soluble and insoluble fibres are two different categories of dietary fibre.

Water

The most prevalent material in the human body is water, which is also a vital ingredient for good health. Water has several important roles in the body, including controlling body temperature, producing bodily fluids, transporting nutrients, and removing waste.

Chapter 2

What to Eat During Pregnancy: A Guide

You should consume more protein, calcium, iron, and important vitamins while you are pregnant. Eat a variety of lean meat, fish, whole grains, and plant-based foods to acquire them.

When creating a healthy eating strategy, you should put focus on whole foods that provide you with more of the nutrients you'd require if you weren't pregnant, like protein, vitamins, and minerals.

Here are 13 nutrient-dense foods you should eat while expecting to help you maintain a healthy diet.

1. Dairy goods

To meet your baby's demands, you'll need more protein and calcium during pregnancy. Dairy items are a wonderful option, including milk, cheese, and yoghurt. Casein and whey are two types of superior protein found in dairy products. The best dietary source of calcium is dairy. Additionally, it supplies magnesium, zinc, phosphorus, and B vitamins. Yoghurt may be especially healthy since it contains probiotic microorganisms that help maintain digestive health.

Yoghurt, especially probiotic yoghurt, may be tolerated by lactose-intolerant people.

2. Legumes

Lentils, peas, beans, chickpeas, soybeans, and peanuts are a few of these. Legumes are excellent plant-based providers of calcium, iron, folate, fibre, protein, and other nutrients that your body needs more of while pregnant.

One of the B vitamins that is most crucial is folate (B9). It is crucial for both you and your unborn child, especially in the first trimester and even earlier.

You must consume at least 600 micrograms (mcg) of folate each day, which can be difficult to do through diet alone. But in addition to supplements, eating more beans might increase your folate levels.

Some legumes are also abundant in iron, magnesium, and potassium, and legumes typically have significant fibre content. Think about including legumes in your diet with dishes like lentil curry, hummus over whole grain toast, and black beans in a taco salad.

3. The sweet potato

Beta-carotene, a plant molecule that your body converts to vitamin A, is abundant in sweet potatoes.

The development of a baby depends on vitamin A. However, consuming too much vitamin A—found in foods like organ meats—can be harmful. A good plant-based source of beta-carotene and fibre is sweet potatoes. Fibre helps you feel fuller for longer, lowers blood sugar surges, and enhances digestive health, all of which can help lower the risk of constipation during pregnancy. When making avocado toast for brunch, try using sweet potatoes as the base.

4. Salmon

Salmon is a nice addition to this list and goes well smoked on a whole wheat bagel, teriyaki grilled, or served with pesto.

Essential omega-3 fatty acids, which offer a wide range of advantages, are abundant in salmon. Fish and seafood contain omega-3s. They may lengthen the gestation period and aid in the development of your baby's brain and eyes.

Salmon, sardines, and anchovies are okay to consume but it's advisable to avoid other seafood while pregnant owing to mercury and other toxins. However, it's important to find out where the fish was caught, especially if it was locally caught. Additionally, choosing fresh salmon is preferred because smoked seafood has a listeria risk.

Swordfish, shark, king mackerel, marlin, bigeye tuna, tilefish from the Gulf of Mexico, and other high-mercury fish should be avoided during pregnancy.

5. Eggs

Eggs are a nutritious food because they have a small amount of practically every vitamin you require. About 71 calories, 3.6 g of protein, fat, and a wealth of vitamins and minerals are found in one large egg. The essential vitamin choline, which is needed during pregnancy, is abundant in eggs. It is crucial for a baby's brain growth and aids in preventing improper brain and spine development.

A single entire egg has about 147 milligrams (mg) of choline, bringing you closer to the current daily choline consumption recommendation of 450 mg when pregnant, though additional research is being done to see whether this is sufficient.

6. Broccoli and leafy, dark vegetables

Many of the nutrients you need are in dark, leafy greens like kale and spinach as well as broccoli. If you don't like the flavours, you can cover them up by putting them in spaghetti sauces, soups, and other dishes. Fibre, vitamin C, vitamin K, vitamin A, calcium, iron, folate, and potassium are all advantages. The fibre in them can aid in preventing constipation. Additionally, vegetables have been associated with a lower risk of low birth weight.

7. Lean proteins and meat

Lean meats like chicken, pork, and beef are great sources of high-quality protein. Iron, choline, and other B vitamins, all of which you'll need in greater amounts when pregnant, are also abundant in beef and pork.

Red blood cells employ iron as a necessary material in the formation of haemoglobin. Since your blood volume is growing, especially in the third trimester, you'll need extra iron. Iron deficiency anaemia may result from low iron levels in the first and second trimesters of pregnancy, which raises the danger of low birth weight and other problems. It may be challenging to meet your iron requirements just through food, particularly if you have a meat allergy or consume only plant-based foods. Lean red meat, on the other hand, might enhance the amount of iron you get from food for those who can.

8. Berries

Berries offer antioxidants, fibre, vitamin C, water, and healthful carbohydrates. Additionally, they have a pretty low glycemic index rating, which means that they shouldn't significantly raise blood sugar levels.

Due to their high water and fibre content, berries make a fantastic snack. They have few calories but offer a lot of flavour and nutrition. Blueberries, raspberries, goji berries, strawberries, and acai berries are some of the greatest berries to consume while expecting.

9. Whole grains

Whole grains have a high amount of fibre, vitamins, and plant components in comparison to their processed cousins. Instead of white bread, spaghetti, and white rice, consider oats, quinoa, brown rice, wheat berries, and barley.

Oats and quinoa are two examples of whole grains that also have a significant amount of protein in addition to B vitamins, fibre, and magnesium.

10. Avocados

The monounsaturated fatty acids are found in avocados. This gives them a buttery, creamy flavour that is ideal for adding depth and creaminess to dishes. Additionally, they offer fibre, anti-oxidants, and B vitamins, including folate, vitamin K, potassium, copper, vitamin E, and vitamin C. Avocados are a fantastic option during pregnancy due to their high levels of good fats, folate, and potassium.

Folate may help prevent neural tube defects and developmental abnormalities of the brain and spine, such as spina bifida, while healthy fats help your child's skin, brain, and tissues develop. Some patients can experience leg cramps, which potassium may help to ease. Bananas and avocados both have more potassium.

11. Stale fruit

In general, dried fruit has a lot of calories, fibre, and different vitamins and minerals. Even though dried fruit is significantly smaller and lacks water, it nevertheless has the same amount of nutrients as fresh fruit.

You can increase your intake of numerous vitamins and minerals, such as folate, iron, and potassium, with just one serving of dried fruit.

Prunes include high levels of potassium, fibre, and vitamin K. They are effective natural laxatives and can aid with constipation. Dates are rich in plant chemicals, potassium, fibre, and iron. However, candied fruit has added sugar in addition to the high levels of natural sugar found in dried fruit.

12. Salmon liver oil

The oily liver of fish, typically from cod, is used to make fish liver oil.

The omega-3 fatty acids EPA and DHA, which are crucial for the growth of the embryonic brain and eyes, are abundant in them.

Taking fish oil supplements may help prevent preterm birth and may be beneficial for the development of the fetus' eyes. A lot of people lack vitamin D, which fish liver oil is abundant in. If you don't typically consume seafood or if you don't currently take vitamin D or omega-3 supplements, it might be helpful.

A tablespoon (4.5 grams) of cod liver oil contains 11 micrograms (mcg), or around 75% of a person's daily needs, of vitamin D and 1,350 mcg, or roughly 150% of a person's daily needs, of vitamin A.

Before using cod liver oil or other omega-3 supplements, see a doctor because taking too much vitamin A or D might be harmful. Additionally, high omega-3 intake may have blood-thinning effects. Pollock, sardines, canned light tuna, and other low-mercury seafood can also help increase omega-3 levels.

13. Water

Everyone needs to stay hydrated, but pregnant women especially need to do so. Blood volume rises by roughly 45% during pregnancy.

To prevent dehydration in both you and your infant, drink plenty of water. Headaches, worry, exhaustion, a negative attitude, and impaired memory are all signs of mild dehydration. Increasing your water intake may also help you avoid urinary tract infections, which are prevalent during pregnancy, and improve constipation.

Chapter 3

Foods That Foster Babies' Health

Your child's body needs certain nutrients from each food group to grow and function effectively. We must therefore consume a variety of meals from all five dietary groups.

Veggies and fruits

Your youngster will gain energy, vitamins, antioxidants, fibre, and water from eating fruit and veggies.

These nutrients work to shield your child from conditions including heart disease, stroke, and some types of cancer in later life.

Offering your infant fruits and vegetables at each meal and as snacks is a smart idea. Try to select fresh and cooked fruits and vegetables with a variety of hues, flavours, and textures.

Fruit should be washed to eliminate any dirt or pesticides and any edible skin should be left on as the skin also has nutrients.

Grain products

Bread, pasta, noodles, morning cereals, couscous, rice, corn, quinoa, polenta, oats, and barley are examples of grain foods. These foods provide kids with the energy they require for learning, development, and growth.

Wholegrain pasta and bread will give your child longer-lasting energy and keep them feeling fuller for longer. These grain foods have low glycaemic indexes.

Dairy

Milk, cheese, and yoghurt are essential dairy products. These meals are excellent providers of calcium and protein.

Dairy foods can be introduced to babies as early as six months. However, until they are about 12 months old when the majority of kids eat meals with their families, make sure that your baby drinks just breastmilk or infant formula. After then, if your child is consuming a healthy diet, you can offer them full-fat cow's milk.

Children in this age range require a lot of energy and rapid growth, thus they require full-fat dairy products until they are two.

Protein

Lean meat, fish, poultry, eggs, beans, lentils, chickpeas, tofu, and nuts are examples of foods high in protein. These nutrients are crucial for your child's development of muscles and growth.

Other beneficial vitamins and minerals like iron, zinc, vitamin B12, and omega-3 fatty acids are also present in these foods. Your child's brain growth and academic success depend primarily on iron and omega-3 fatty acids from red meat and oily seafood.

Healthy beverages

The healthiest beverage for children over the age of one year is water. The cost is also the lowest. Fluoride is typically added to tap water to strengthen teeth as well.

Breastfed and formula-fed infants can begin drinking small amounts of cooled, boiling tap water from a cup at six months of age.

Restricted foods and beverages

It's best to restrict how much sometimes food your youngster consumes. This implies that your youngster will have more space for regular, healthy diets.

Fast food, takeout, and junk food like hot chips, potato chips, dim sum, pies, burgers, and takeout pizza are examples of "sometimes" foods. Additionally, cakes, chocolate, candies, biscuits, doughnuts, and pastries are among these items.

Chapter 4

Avoiding Certain Foods and Drinks While Pregnant

In general, foods that increase the risk of infection during pregnancy should be avoided, such as undercooked or raw meat or fish, but you should also limit your intake of caffeine and processed meals.

To properly nourish yourself and your unborn child throughout pregnancy, consume a healthy diet. Some of your favourite foods, like sushi, coffee, or rare steak, might have to be given up.

Following are 15 foods and drinks to avoid or consume in moderation when pregnant:

1. Mercury-rich fish

The highly hazardous metal mercury can be found in contaminated waters. It can have an impact on your kidneys, immunological system, and brain system in higher doses. Children who consume it may also experience major developmental issues; harmful effects can still occur at smaller doses.

Large marine fish should be avoided during pregnancy and breastfeeding because they can collect large quantities of mercury.

Sharks, swordfish, king mackerel, tuna (particularly bigeye tuna), and marlin are high-mercury species to stay away from.

2. Raw or undercooked fish

There is a significant chance that raw fish, particularly shellfish, will have germs or parasites like norovirus, Vibrio, Salmonella, or Listeria.

During handling, storing, and processing, such as smoking or drying, raw fish might get an infection. Even if you don't experience any symptoms, some of these infections can travel via the placenta to your baby and cause dehydration and weakness in the parents. They can raise the chance of premature labour, miscarriage, stillbirth, and other life-threatening medical issues. Pregnancy increases the risk of listeria infection by up to

10 times compared to other periods of the year.

3. Raw or undercooked meat

Eating meat that is undercooked or uncooked increases your chance of contracting bacteria or parasites like Toxoplasma or E. Salmonella, E. coli, and Listeria. Both your health and the health and safety of your child could be in danger from bacteria.

The majority of germs are found on the surface of complete chunks of meat, however, some may persist within the muscle fibres. Tenderloins, sirloins, and ribeye from beef, lamb, and veal are some entire cuts of meat that may be safe to eat even when not fully cooked. This is true only if the meat is entire or uncut and has finished cooking on the outside.

It's advised to stay away from any undercooked meat when pregnant. It is never advisable to consume cut meat that is raw or undercooked, including beef patties, burgers, minced meat, pig, and chicken.

4. Deli meat and processed meat

During preparation or storage, several bacteria can contaminate hot dogs, lunch meat, pepperoni, and deli meat. Because they are not cooked, cured meats could contain bacteria or parasites. Furthermore, processed meats may be heavy in sodium and harmful fats. It is recommended to stay away from deli meats and make sure that processed meats you cook, like sausages, are well-cooked.

5. A raw egg

Salmonella bacteria can be found in raw eggs. Salmonella infections can cause fever, nausea, vomiting, pains in the stomach, and diarrhoea. Additionally, it could result in uterine cramping, which might result in a stillbirth or preterm birth.

Lightly scrambled eggs, tiramisu, raw batter, hollandaise sauce, homemade mayonnaise, some salad dressings, homemade egg nog, handmade ice cream, some homemade cake icings, and eggs Benedict are a few examples of foods that frequently contain raw eggs.

The majority of commercially available raw egg products are manufactured with pasteurized eggs and are safe to eat. Use pasteurized eggs or be sure to properly boil your eggs.

6. Flesh from organs

Organ meats include a variety of vital elements that are healthy for both you and your unborn child, including iron, vitamin B12, vitamin A, zinc, selenium, and copper.

Pregnant women should avoid taking excessive amounts of preformed vitamin A because it can cause birth defects and miscarriage.

It's preferable to consume only a few ounces of meats like liver or kidney every week, even though this is generally related to vitamin A supplements.

7. Fresh sprouts

Alfalfa, clover, radish, and mung bean sprouts are among the common raw sprouts used in salads. Salmonella can grow best in the humid atmosphere that seeds require to begin sprouting, and it is nearly tough to remove. Because of this, it's recommended to stay away from raw sprouts completely, while they're fine to eat cooked.

8. Fresh produce that hasn't been washed

Fruits and vegetables that have not been washed or peeled may have germs and parasites like Toxoplasma on their surface. Listeria, Salmonella, and E. coli. These might be acquired through handling or from the soil. During production, harvest, processing, storage, transportation, or retail, contamination can happen at any time.

A parasite called toxoplasma can survive on plant-based diets. The majority of people don't have any symptoms, but the parasite can pass through the placenta and lead to eyesight loss and learning challenges in later life.

Some babies may be born with significant eye or brain impairment.

All fruits and vegetables should be well-cleaned with fresh water before eating to reduce the danger of illness.

9. Dairy products without pasteurization

Listeria, Salmonella, and other dangerous bacteria can be found in raw milk and other unpasteurized dairy products. as well as Campylobacter. These bacteria have the potential to cause a variety of diseases known as food poisoning.

All of these infections have the potential to be fatal to an unborn child.

The bacteria may develop naturally or as a result of collection or storage site contamination. Any hazardous bacteria can be eliminated by pasteurization without affecting the nutritional content of the goods. Eat only pasteurized dairy products to lower your risk of illnesses.

10. Supple cheeses

Listeria, a type of bacteria that can lead to serious illness and miscarriage, is present in several soft cheeses. The following are some examples: queso ranchero, panela, blando, blanco, and fresco. Eat soft cheeses only if the label indicates that they have been pasteurized.

11. Packaged food

Low in nutrition, rich in calories, sugar, and added fats, highly processed foods may raise the risk of weight gain.

You need to consume enough protein, folate, choline, and iron when you're pregnant. In addition, while some weight growth is required, excessive weight gain raises the risk of both childhood obesity and delivery problems.

Keep your meals and snacks focused on protein, fruits and vegetables, whole grains, legumes, and starchy vegetables that are high in fibre. Discover some fresh approaches to including vegetables in your meals without compromising flavour.

12. Several fruit smoothies and liquids

Fruit juices can be helpful during pregnancy, but choose pasteurized juices without added sugar. Raw juices, such as those made at market stalls, may have dangerous bacteria in them. Unpasteurized juice can be found in smoothies as well.

13. Alcohol

Alcohol consumption during pregnancy raises the risk of fetal alcohol syndrome (FAS), stillbirth, and pregnancy loss. Heart and brain development are only two of the many areas of development that FAS can impact. It's best to stay away from alcohol completely because there is no known safe amount to consume while pregnant.

14. Caffeine

Caffeine can be found in coffee, tea, soft drinks, and chocolate. A high caffeine intake increases the chance of miscarriage, stillbirth, low birth weight, and different developmental problems. The placenta may easily absorb caffeine and it is swiftly absorbed by the body. High quantities of caffeine can accumulate because newborns and their placentas lack the primary enzyme required for its metabolization.

15. Contaminated water for drinking

To prevent dehydration during pregnancy, you must consume plenty of water. Although the majority of tap water is safe to consume, chemicals in dirty or polluted water can harm you or your unborn child. If you utilize water from a private well, this can apply to you.

Chapter 5

Nutritional Supplements

A manufactured substance known as a dietary supplement can be taken as a pill, capsule, tablet, powder, or liquid to complement your diet. To boost the amount of nutrients consumed, a supplement can include either synthetic or nutrients that have been derived from dietary sources. Vitamins, minerals, fibre, fatty acids, and amino acids are among the group of nutritional molecules.

Additionally, dietary supplements may contain ingredients like plant pigments or polyphenols that are touted as having positive biological effects but have not been proven to be necessary for survival. Ingredients for supplements can also come from animals, such as fish or chicken collagen. These can be blended with nutritious substances and are also sold alone and in sets.

Vitamins

A vitamin is an organic substance that an organism needs in little amounts as a critical nutrient. When an organism is unable to produce an organic chemical molecule in sufficient quantities and must instead acquire it from the diet, it is referred to as a vitamin. The phrase is dependent on both the environment and the specific creature. For instance, anthropoid monkeys, humans, guinea pigs, and bats all require ascorbic acid (vitamin C), although other animals do not. For those who receive enough UV radiation from the sun or an artificial source to synthesise vitamin D in their skin, vitamin D is not a necessary nutrient. Thirteen vitamins are necessary for human nutrition, the majority of which are actually "vitamers"—groups of related molecules—(for example, vitamin E contains tocopherols and tocotrienols, while vitamin K contains vitamins K1 and K2).

Vitamins A, C, D, E, K, Thiamine, Riboflavin, Niacin, Pantothenic Acid,

Vitamin B6, Biotin, Folate, and Vitamin B12 are included in the list. Vitamin consumption that is below the required levels might cause the signs and symptoms of vitamin insufficiency. There is minimal proof that taking vitamins as dietary supplements can help people who are healthy and eat a balanced diet.

Minerals

The external chemical elements required for life are minerals. Four minerals—carbon, hydrogen, oxygen, and nitrogen—are necessary for life but are present in so many foods and beverages that they are not regarded as nutrients and do not have recommended daily intakes. The requirements for protein, which is made up of amino acids that include nitrogen, are intended to address the need for nitrogen. Despite being necessary for humans, there is no specific suggested intake for sulfur. The amino acids methionine and cysteine, which contain sulfur, have suggested intakes instead. Sulfur can be found in dietary supplements like taurine and methylsulfonylmethane.

Proteins

Protein-rich supplements are marketed as aids for those recovering from illness or injury, those hoping to prevent the sarcopenia of old age, athletes who believe that strenuous exercise increases protein requirements, those hoping to lose weight while minimizing muscle loss, i.e., conducting a protein-sparing modified fast, and those hoping to increase muscle size for performance. In addition to casein, soy, pea, hemp, and rice protein, goods may also contain the widely used ingredient whey protein. Whey protein supplements are a safe and effective addition to an athlete's training and recovery, according to a meta-analysis, which also indicated benefits for muscle mass, endurance, average power, and decreased perceived exercise intensity.

Supplements for bodybuilders

Bodybuilding supplements are dietary additives that are frequently consumed by people who engage in bodybuilding, weightlifting, mixed martial arts, and athletics to promote the growth of lean body mass. Ingredients in bodybuilding supplements may be claimed to improve muscle mass, body weight, athletic performance, and body fat percentage for desired muscular definition. High protein beverages, pre-workout mixtures, branched-chain amino acids (BCAA), glutamine, arginine, essential fatty acids, creatine, HMB, whey protein, ZMA, and weight loss products are a few of the most popular.

Supplements can be purchased as single-ingredient formulations or as "stacks"—proprietary combinations of many supplements that are touted as having synergistic effects.

Important fatty acids

Because it contains omega-3 fatty acids, fish oil is a popular fatty acid supplement. Carbon atoms are strung together to form fatty acids, which can vary in length. A fatty acid is referred described as "saturated" if all of its bonds are single (C-C); "monounsaturated" if only one of its bonds is double (C=C); and "polyunsaturated" refers to two or more double bonds (C=C=C).

Since the body can make the other fatty acids, just two essential polyunsaturated fatty acids are thought to need to be consumed through diet.

The "essential" fatty acids are linoleic acid (LA), an omega-6 fatty acid, and alpha-linolenic acid (ALA), an omega-3 fatty acid.

Eicosapentaenoic acid (EPA) and docosahexaenoic acid (DHA) are two additional omega-3 fatty acids that can be produced in the body by elongating ALA.

All-natural goods

Ginkgo biloba, curcumin, cranberries, St. John's wort, ginseng, resveratrol, glucosamine, and collagen are just a few examples of the types of natural ingredients that can be used to make dietary supplements. Without a prescription, products with advertising claims of health advantages are sold at pharmacies, supermarkets, speciality stores, military commissaries, buyers' clubs, direct selling organizations, and online. Although the majority of these products have a lengthy history of usage in herbalism and different types of traditional medicine.

Probiotics

Probiotic supplement claims are not sufficiently validated by clinical research. Children taking probiotics show a slight decrease in acute diarrhoea and antibiotic-associated diarrhoea, according to meta-analysis research. For the relief of irritable bowel syndrome symptoms in adults, there is very weak evidence to support the use of mono- and multi-strain probiotics. Supplements with probiotics are typically thought to be secure.

Fertility

Men who took supplements containing selenium, zinc, omega-3 fatty acids, coenzyme Q10, or carnitines reported improvements in total sperm count, concentration, motility, and morphology, according to preliminary research from a meta-analysis. According to a review, infertile men may have improved semen quality if they consume omega-3 through supplements and diet. However, it cautioned that "excessive use of antioxidants may be detrimental to the spermatic function" and that "many of the over-the-counter supplements are not

scientifically proven to improve fertility."
A 2021 review also endorsed selenium, zinc, omega-3 fatty acids, coenzyme Q10, or carnitines.

Prenatal

To provide pregnant women with nutrients that may lessen health concerns for both the mother and fetus, prenatal vitamins are frequently administered as dietary supplements.

Prenatal supplementation may be helpful for pregnant women at risk of nutrient deficiencies due to food constraints or restrictions, even though prenatal vitamins are not meant to replace dietary nutrition.

Vitamins B6, folate, B12, C, D, E, iron, and calcium are among the prenatal vitamins that typically contain these ingredients.

A sufficient dose of vitamin B6 helps ease morning sickness symptoms and reduce the risk of early pregnancy loss. For pregnant women to avoid neural tube abnormalities, folate is also a crucial nutrient. The World Health Organization recommended in 2006 that women of childbearing age have 400 micrograms of folate daily from their diets if they were considering getting pregnant.

According to a 2013 review, using folic acid supplements during pregnancy had no other effects on the mother's health outside lowering the risk of megaloblastic anemia and low pre-delivery serum folate.

www.ingramcontent.com/pod-product-compliance
Lightning Source LLC
Chambersburg PA
CBHW061522250726

48657CB00005B/2012